FROM MANAGING TO CONQUERING DANDRUFF

Expert Guide To Understanding Causes, Identifying Symptoms, And Implementing Effective Treatments For A Scalp-Soothing Journey To Healthy Living

DR. DASHIELL DANIEL

ABOUT THIS BOOK

The book "DANDRUFF" provides a thorough examination of the complex phenomenon of dandruff and is an invaluable tool for anybody looking for a deeper comprehension of this widespread scalp ailment. This book is significant because it takes a methodical approach to deciphering the complexities of dandruff and combines scientific understanding with useful advice for efficient care. Through an exploration of the basic causes of dandruff, the book provides readers with the information they need to make wise choices about preventative and treatment options.

The book provides a basic grasp of dandruff in the introduction, dispelling myths and preparing the reader for a thorough investigation. The following chapters explore the scientific basis of dandruff, explaining the complex structure of the scalp, the workings of the dandruff cycle, and the variables that contribute to its appearance.

The book goes on to categorize dandruff into different forms, covering variations for both oily and dry scalps. Through the provision of comprehensive insights into the symptoms, etiology, and efficacious treatment modalities associated with each kind, readers get a sophisticated comprehension that enables tailored approaches to the management of their particular ailment. The book's emphasis on self-evaluation and obtaining expert advice highlights its dedication to providing readers with the resources required for precise identification and individualized care.

Chapters on over-the-counter medications, herbal therapies, and lifestyle changes provide a comprehensive approach to managing dandruff. The comprehensive material on dietary modifications, stress management, and herbal remedies is included in the book, which further emphasizes its dedication to examining a wide range of strategies. Furthermore, the book's examination of cutting-edge remedies including prescription drugs and light therapy demonstrates its dedication to offering up-to-date knowledge on managing dandruff.

The last few chapters discuss the critical topic of avoiding dandruff recurrence, providing long-term solutions and stressing the value of keeping the scalp healthy. The emphasis on maintaining a balanced scalp microbiome and scheduling routine examinations highlights the book's dedication to treating current dandruff while also encouraging long-term scalp health.

Essentially, "DANDRUFF" becomes an indispensable tool that bridges the gap between scientific understanding and real-world application. Its importance comes from its comprehensive and subtle approach, which makes it a valuable resource for anyone trying to accurately and intelligently traverse the complications of dandruff.

Introduction

People who want to have the healthiest possible hair and scalp have always been concerned about dandruff, a frequent ailment of the scalp. In order to effectively manage dandruff, it is important to understand its nuances, including its definition, causes, and frequent myths that should be cleared up.

Recognizing Dandruff

The dermatological disorder known as dandruff is typified by the exfoliation of dead skin cells from the scalp, frequently accompanied by discomfort and itching. Although the specific cause of it is unknown, a number of factors influence how it manifests. Dandruff is intimately associated with a common skin ailment called seborrheic dermatitis. Furthermore, the growth of dandruff has been linked to a fungus called Malassezia that lives on the scalp and resembles yeast.

The way these elements interact leads to an atmosphere that promotes inflammation and higher cell turnover, which produces the noticeable flakes connected to dandruff.

Typical Myths

Despite being common, dandruff is sometimes misunderstood, which makes treatment difficult. One popular misconception is that bad hygiene is the only thing that causes dandruff.

While frequent hair washing is necessary, overdoing it can make the problem worse by depriving the scalp of its natural oils, which makes the skin flakier and drier. The idea that dandruff is contagious is another myth.

Despite popular assumption, dandruff is not a contagious disease; rather, it is the consequence of a complex interplay of genetic, environmental, and personal variables. Clearing up these misunderstandings is essential to creating focused and knowledgeable dandruff-fighting techniques.

Reasons For Dandruff

Developing successful management strategies for dandruff requires a thorough understanding of its complex causes. One of the main causes is seborrheic dermatitis, a chronic inflammatory disease. Skin cell shedding increases as a result of its disruption of the regular function of the skin barrier. Malassezia is another important player; it's a naturally occurring yeast on the scalp.

It interacts with sebum, the natural oil of the skin, to cause an inflammatory reaction that speeds up skin cell turnover. Furthermore, dandruff growth is influenced by personal factors such as hormonal changes, stress, and specific medical problems. Developing solutions that target the underlying causes requires an understanding of the complex interactions between these variables.

Microbiota On The Scalp And Dandruff

A variety of microorganisms known as the scalp microbiome are essential to the health of the scalp and the development of dandruff.

A well-known microbiome component called Malassezia has been linked to the pathophysiology of dandruff. It breaks down sebum to produce oleic acid, which can irritate the scalp and weaken its protective layer.

Comprehending the intricate correlation between the scalp microbiome and dandruff offers valuable perspectives on possible therapies that aim to balance the microbial population.

In order to modify the scalp microbiome, create a healthy atmosphere, and lessen the symptoms of dandruff, probiotics and antibacterial medications may prove to be useful tools.

Techniques Of Management

Dandruff can only be effectively conquered with a complete strategy that takes care of the underlying causes as well as the symptoms.

Topical antifungal medications that target Malassezia and reduce inflammation include ketoconazole and selenium sulfide. Using specific shampoos on a regular basis and gently can help control problems.

But it's important to find a balance because too much washing might make things worse. Stressing a healthy, nutrient-rich diet promotes scalp health generally and addresses dietary inadequacies that may be a factor in dandruff. There are situations where lowering stress through lifestyle changes and relaxation methods can also help lessen the intensity of dandruff.

New Research And Therapies

Research developments in dermatology are still illuminating novel treatments for dandruff. Personalized medicine methods that take into account each patient's unique genetic and microbiological makeup have the potential to improve the efficacy of interventions.

Research is still being done to find innovative antifungal drugs that specifically target Malassezia without affecting the healthy elements of the scalp microbiome.

In the future, developing a better understanding of the genetic basis of dandruff susceptibility may lead to gene-based therapeutics. The field of dandruff management is expected to change as research advances, bringing with it more accurate and practical remedies.

Fighting dandruff requires a comprehensive knowledge of its underlying causes, busting myths, and using all-encompassing management techniques.

There are many factors to consider on the path to efficient dandruff treatment, from the complexities of the scalp microbiome to newly developed medicinal strategies.

People may manage the complexity of dandruff and obtain healthier, flake-free scalps by fusing scientific findings with doable solutions.

CHAPTER ONE
THE SCIENCE OF DANDRUFF
Anatomy Of The Scalp

The human scalp, a dynamic and intricate structure, is a major contributor to the development of dandruff. The scalp has a multilayered structure, with the epidermis, the outermost layer, being particularly significant. This layer constantly renews itself, removing old skin cells to make room for new ones. Hair follicles and blood vessels are found in the dermis, the innermost layer, which helps to nourish and grow hair. Insulation and support are given by the subcutaneous tissue located beneath the dermis.

The Scale's Layers Are

The three primary layers of the scalp are the subcutaneous tissue, dermis, and epidermis.

The outermost layer, the epidermis, acts as a barrier to protect the skin from outside influences. The dermis has blood vessels, nerves, and hair follicles underneath it. The innermost layer, the subcutaneous tissue, is insulated and contains fat cells.

Comprehending the formation of dandruff and its efficient management requires an understanding of these layers.

Sebaceous Glands And Hair Follicles

Hair growth depends on the hair follicles that are dispersed across the scalp. Sebaceous glands, which produce sebum, an oily fluid that hydrates and shields the hair and scalp, are attached to each hair follicle. Dandruff may arise as a result of these glands producing an excessive amount of sebum. Furthermore, the clogged hair follicles might create an environment that is favorable to the formation of Malassezia, the yeast-like fungus linked to dandruff.

The Cycle Of Dandruff

Comprehending the cycle of dandruff is essential for tackling its underlying causes. On the scalp, skin cells are constantly renewing themselves as part of this cycle. Old cells shed when they die, allowing way for new ones to grow.

Yet, this process is sped up in people who are prone to dandruff, resulting in the production of noticeable flakes. The presence of specific microorganisms on the scalp or an excessive immune response are two common conditions that accompany the uneven shedding of skin cells.

How Dandruff Flakes Form

Dead skin cells make up the majority of dandruff flakes. On the scalp, these cells shed more quickly, leaving behind noticeable white or yellow-colored flakes. Environmental influences, genetic predisposition, and hormone fluctuations all have an impact on this process.

Furthermore, increased oleic acid synthesis is frequently linked to the expansion of Malassezia, a naturally occurring yeast on the scalp, which can cause inflammation and aid in the development of dandruff flakes.

Factors Associated With Dandruff

Dandruff is a complex disorder that develops as a result of multiple circumstances. Hormonal changes can affect sebum production and exacerbate dandruff, particularly in adolescence. Another factor is genetic predisposition; people who have a family history of dandruff may be more prone.

Dry and flaky hair can result from environmental causes like cold, dry weather that deplete the scalp's natural oils. Additionally, dandruff can develop or worsen as a result of stress, decreased immunity, and other medical disorders.

the science underlying dandruff is complex and requires a deep comprehension of the anatomy of the scalp, the dandruff cycle, and the variables that contribute to the development of dandruff. Dandruff management and prevention require a comprehensive strategy that takes into account both internal and environmental influences.

CHAPTER TWO
DANDRUFF TYPES

A common scalp condition called dandruff can take many different forms, each of which requires a deeper understanding in order to effectively treat. One common kind is called "dry scalp dandruff," which is defined by the scalp's dry skin flaking off. People who have this illness frequently detect tiny, white flakes in their hair and clothes.

Dandruff on a dry scalp frequently comes with itching and discomfort. Cold temperatures, low humidity, and the use of harsh hair care products that deplete the scalp of its natural oils can all contribute to this kind of dandruff. A focused skincare regimen and treating the underlying causes are two effective treatments for dandruff on a dry scalp. Dryness can be relieved temporarily by moisturizing the scalp with natural oils like coconut oil. Long-term treatment can be achieved by avoiding harsh shampoos and choosing ones with hydrating components instead.

A balanced diet high in vitamins and minerals can also help to maintain the health of the scalp and lessen the chance of developing dry scalp dandruff.

On the other hand, greasy scalp dandruff poses a distinct set of difficulties, as it is defined by an overabundance of oil production resulting in the buildup of oily, yellowish flakes on the scalp. Effective management of oily scalp dandruff requires an understanding of its causes.

Genetics, hormone imbalances, and an overactive sebaceous gland are some of the factors that might cause excessive oil output.

It is crucial to have a focused strategy that tackles both the excessive oil production and the flaking that results in order to treat oily scalp dandruff. Utilizing specialty shampoos with components like zinc pyrithione, ketoconazole, or salicylic acid might help reduce oil production and fight the fungus growth that is frequently linked to dandruff. Regularly washing the scalp with these shampoos and avoiding thick, oil-based hair products can help maintain a healthier environment on the scalp. Additionally, controlling sebum production and promoting general scalp health can be achieved by implementing a well-balanced diet that includes zinc and omega-3 fatty acids.

Although there are two different forms of scalp dandruff—oily and dry—it's important to understand that people can have both, necessitating a thorough treatment plan.

For successful outcomes in these situations, a customized treatment strategy that addresses both dryness and excess oil production is necessary. Furthermore, managing and preventing dandruff requires adhering to basic hygiene measures, such as routinely washing the hair and scalp. People may choose products and hair care routines more intelligently when they are aware of the unique traits and underlying reasons of each type of dandruff.

treating dandruff effectively necessitates having a solid awareness of its several forms, each of which requires a different strategy. Dry scalp dandruff necessitates a well-balanced skincare routine with an emphasis on moisturizing due to its characteristic white flakes and irritation. Oily scalp dandruff, which is characterized by greasy, yellowish flakes, requires specific shampoos and a focused cleaning routine to regulate overproduction of oil. Understanding how oiliness and dryness interact is critical for people who experience both at the same time. People can effectively treat and avoid dandruff, a common scalp ailment, by using a holistic approach that tackles the specific characteristics and underlying causes of the condition. This promotes general scalp health and well-being.

CHAPTER THREE
DETERMINING THE KIND OF DANDRUFF

Self-Assessment: A comprehensive knowledge of the various expressions of dandruff is necessary. Dandruff is a common scalp problem that is characterized by flaking and itching.

One of the most important initial steps to effective management is self-assessment. Seeing symptoms entails closely inspecting the scalp for indications including redness, itching, and white or yellow flakes. The size and structure of the flakes can reveal information about how severe the illness is. In contrast to oily dandruff, which is typified by bigger, yellowish flakes that frequently stick to the scalp and hair, dry dandruff is characterized by tiny, white flakes. Knowing these differences makes it easier to customize a suitable treatment plan.

Recognizing Triggers: There are several factors that contribute to dandruff, which is a complex disorder. Potential contributions can be identified by carefully examining lifestyle, nutrition, and environmental factors. Dandruff can be made worse by specific food choices, stress, and poor hair care practices. Environmental elements that can also have an impact include humidity levels and exposure to harsh hair products. Being aware of these triggers enables people to choose appropriate scalp care products and make educated lifestyle choices. The incidence and intensity of dandruff episodes can be greatly decreased by recognizing and addressing triggers.

Looking For Expert Advice

Dermatological Consultations: In order to fully comprehend dandruff, professional advice must be sought, even though self-evaluation might yield insightful information. Consultations with dermatologists provide a more thorough examination of the scalp problem. Dermatologists can accurately diagnose patients because of their specific knowledge, which allows them to distinguish between different scalp problems.

They take into account variables including lifestyle, family history, and medical history to offer a comprehensive understanding of the root causes of dandruff. Additionally, dermatologists can create individualized treatment programs that combine lifestyle advice with medication procedures for the best possible outcomes.

Diagnostic testing: To accurately determine the underlying reasons of dandruff, doctors may occasionally advise diagnostic testing. To identify the precise microorganisms causing the ailment, these procedures could involve fungal cultures, microscopic analyses, and scalp biopsies.

Tests for diagnosis are especially helpful if the dandruff is severe, chronic, or resistant to standard therapies. By employing a methodical approach, dermatologists can identify latent causes of dandruff, like fungal infections or inflammatory diseases, allowing for focused and efficient treatment. Getting the diagnosis right is essential to creating a customized treatment plan that targets the underlying causes of dandruff.

To sum up, treating dandruff requires a complete knowledge of the ailment, beginning with determining its type via self-evaluation.

The foundation of this procedure is observing symptoms and identifying triggers, which directs people toward customized interventions.

Getting expert advice improves dandruff management even more. Dermatological consultations provide knowledgeable insights, and diagnostic testing is accurate in pinpointing underlying causes. By preventing future recurrences and ensuring the relief of symptoms, this holistic approach promotes the health of the scalp and overall well-being.

CHAPTER FOUR
OVER-THE-COUNTER SOLUTIONS

Many people suffer from dandruff, a common scalp ailment that can cause irritation, flaking, and occasionally humiliation. Solutions available over-the-counter offer a convenient and efficient way to deal with this problem. As the first line of defense, dandruff-specific shampoos are widely accessible and effective.

Shampoos For Cradle Cap

Shampoos designed specifically to address dandruff are essential in the fight against flaky scalps. Typically, the active components in these formulations are used to fight against the overgrowth of Malassezia, a yeast-like fungus that is known to cause dandruff. These specialty shampoos often contain coal tar, ketoconazole, selenium sulfide, and pyridinium zinc as main components.

For instance, pyrithione zinc inhibits the growth of yeast on the scalp, whereas ketoconazole acts as an antifungal medication by going straight after the Malassezia fungus. Coal tar and selenium sulfide work by slowing down skin cell growth, which stops the rapid shedding of skin cells that causes dandruff.

Selecting The Appropriate Product

When choosing the best dandruff shampoo, it's important to take into account things like your skin type, the severity of your issue, and any potential sensitivities. It is essential to closely examine product labels in order to determine the concentrations and active components. Furthermore, seeking advice from a dermatologist or other healthcare expert can assist in identifying the best course of action depending on the unique requirements of the patient.

For best effects, use it frequently, a few times a week, and be patient as changes might not show up right away.

Conditioners As Well As Topical Remedies

Apart from shampoos specifically designed to combat dandruff, conditioners and topical treatments are essential for controlling and averting the recurrence of this prevalent scalp problem. Moisturizing methods are especially crucial because they help with the dryness that dandruff frequently causes.

Methods Of Moisturization

Dandruff is frequently accompanied by dryness, and moisturizing the scalp can greatly reduce flakiness and pain. Conditioners designed especially for dry and damaged hair can give the scalp and hair strands the much-needed moisture they require. These conditioners frequently include glycerin, shea butter, and other natural oils that combine to seal in moisture and enhance the general health of the scalp.

Frequent use of a moisturizing conditioner can help create a healthy environment on the scalp, which lowers the chance of dandruff returning.

Products That Are Left Over

Apart from conventional conditioners, leave-in treatments provide a focused method of hydrating the hair. You can apply leave-in conditioners, serums, or oils directly to the scalp and hair to get continuous hydration all day. Ingredients with moisturizing and calming qualities including jojoba oil, argan oil, and aloe vera may be present in these products. Make sure the leave-in product you select is non-comedogenic and safe for your scalp. Certain leave-in formulas might clog pores or worsen the symptoms of dandruff.

A comprehensive approach to dandruff management and scalp health promotion can benefit from the inclusion of leave-in products in a regular hair care regimen.

over-the-counter remedies provide a comprehensive strategy for overcoming dandruff. Shampoos are the first line of defense because their main ingredients work to address the underlying causes of the problem. Selecting the appropriate product necessitates carefully weighing each unique circumstance and consulting medical experts. Conditioners and topical treatments that prioritize moisturizing methods increase the efficacy of the entire plan even more. People can make great progress in controlling dandruff and preserving a healthy scalp environment by treating dryness and feeding the scalp with appropriate treatments on a regular basis.

CHAPTER FIVE
HERBAL CURE
Herbal Remedies

Dandruff is one of many health conditions for which herbal treatments have long been sought for due to their potential. Aloe Vera and Tea Tree Oil are very good at treating this frequent ailment of the scalp. Known for its calming qualities, aloe vera aids in lowering dandruff-related irritation and itching. Its antifungal and antibacterial qualities also support a healthy scalp by preventing the growth of the yeast that frequently causes dandruff. Melaleuca alternifolia leaves are used to make tea tree oil, which is well known for having antifungal and antibacterial properties. It aids in regulating the overgrowth of skin cells on the scalp, which is a major contributor to the development of dandruff. When combined, aloe vera and tea tree oil offer a powerful natural remedy for people with chronic dandruff.

Two fragrant plants that are frequently seen in gardens, rosemary and lavender, are also essential for treating dandruff. Antioxidant and anti-inflammatory qualities are well-known for rosemary. It can increase blood flow to the scalp through topical application or infusion into hair care products, which can encourage hair growth and lessen dandruff. In addition to its soothing aroma, lavender has antibacterial qualities that support a healthy scalp environment. Its calming properties can help reduce the irritation caused by dandruff, which makes it an important supplement to herbal remedies. By utilizing the natural ability of herbs to support healthy scalp function, hair care regimens can effectively manage dandruff in a comprehensive way.

Nutritional Adjustments

Apart from physical remedies, dietary modifications are crucial in managing issues related to dandruff. Certain meals have the ability to either worsen or improve the circumstances that cause dandruff. Foods high in omega-3 fatty acids, such as walnuts, flaxseeds, and salmon, are good for a healthy scalp. Because of their anti-inflammatory qualities, omega-3 fatty acids may help lessen scalp irritation, which is frequently a sign of dandruff. Consuming fruits and vegetables strong in antioxidants can also help maintain the general health of the scalp. Citrus fruits, leafy greens, and berries all include vital vitamins and minerals that support a healthy, well-nourished scalp and lessen the chance of developing dandruff.

Not to be disregarded, hydration and dandruff are related factors in scalp health. Staying well hydrated is crucial for preserving the health of the skin, particularly the scalp. Dandruff symptoms can be made worse by dehydration, which can cause dryness and flakiness. Drinking enough water keeps the skin hydrated from the inside out, which lowers the chance of developing dandruff. Additionally, water promotes the general well-being of hair follicles, which results in hair that is stronger and more resilient. Combining dietary modifications that emphasize staying hydrated—such as eating more fruits and vegetables high in water—with topical treatments and herbal remedies completes a holistic strategy for overcoming dandruff.

achieving hair free of dandruff necessitates a multifaceted strategy that goes beyond traditional remedies. Herbal remedies, which include the medicinal qualities of Aloe Vera, Tea Tree Oil, Rosemary, and Lavender, provide a healthy substitute for goods that contain chemicals.

These herbs relieve symptoms and support healthy scalp function by addressing the underlying causes of dandruff. In addition, dietary modifications—with an emphasis on foods high in antioxidants, omega-3 fatty acids, and sufficient hydration—are essential for controlling and avoiding dandruff. A holistic approach that incorporates dietary changes and natural therapies can help people effectively combat dandruff and keep their scalps healthy.

CHAPTER SIX
ADJUSTMENTS TO LIFESTYLE
Handling Stress

Since stress is closely related to the onset and aggravation of this widespread scalp ailment, managing stress effectively is essential to beating dandruff. Biochemical, psychological, and environmental factors interact in a complicated way to cause dandruff and stress. Persistent stress causes changes in hormones, particularly elevated cortisol levels, which can be detrimental to scalp and skin health in general. Moreover, stress weakens the immune system, increasing the scalp's vulnerability to fungi like Malassezia, which is frequently responsible for the development of dandruff.

People who suffer from stress-related dandruff can use a variety of relaxing methods. These methods include both mental and physical practices, such as progressive muscle relaxation, yoga, and deep breathing exercises in addition to meditation. These activities enhance general wellbeing in addition to reducing stress. For example, studies on meditation have shown that it lowers cortisol levels and boosts immunity, which helps to mitigate the variables that cause dandruff.

A thorough strategy for treating dandruff may include incorporating these stress-reduction measures into one's everyday routine.

Hair Care Routines: Selecting The Ideal Hairbrush

A key component of managing dandruff effectively is choosing the right hairbrush. The impact of various hairbrush materials and designs vary on the scalp and hair. Brushes with widely spaced, rounded bristles are best for people whose scalps are prone to dandruff because they reduce irritation and unnecessary scratching, both of which can worsen the condition. Furthermore, using brushes with natural materials—like boar bristles—can aid in distributing natural oils uniformly throughout the scalp, avoiding dryness, which is sometimes the first sign of dandruff.

On the other hand, brushes composed of synthetic materials or featuring closely spaced, sharp bristles may injure the scalp and increase the symptoms of dandruff. Frequent hairbrush cleaning is also necessary since gathered product residue, oils, and dead skin cells can serve as a haven for the yeast that causes dandruff. People can make a major contribution to the treatment and prevention of dandruff by being mindful of the type of hairbrush they use and keeping it clean.

Washing Methods And Frequency

When managing dandruff, hair washing technique and frequency are crucial factors to take into account. Finding the ideal balance is crucial since problems related to dandruff can arise from both excessive and insufficient shampooing.

For example, overwashing can deplete the scalp of its natural oils, making it drier and more prone to dandruff. However, infrequent washing promotes the buildup of sebum, dead skin cells, and product residues, which in turn fosters the growth of fungi that cause dandruff.

Selecting the right shampoo is just as crucial.

To effectively reduce fungal growth on the scalp, anti-dandruff shampoos with active chemicals such pyrithione zinc, ketoconazole, or selenium sulfide are used. Finding a balance between avoiding dandruff and preserving the health of your scalp can be achieved by using these shampoos sparingly and according to the stated usage instructions. Furthermore, massaging the scalp while showering can improve blood flow and create a more hygienic environment on the scalp.

People can prevent dandruff and promote a healthier scalp by washing their hair as often as possible and with the right methods.

CHAPTER SEVEN
SOPHISTICATED THERAPIES

Common scalp conditions like dandruff can often be treated with over-the-counter shampoos; however, in more severe situations, more sophisticated treatments can be required. Prescription drugs and light therapy are discussed in this section as advanced methods of treating dandruff.

Prescription Drugs

The use of prescription drugs is essential for treating severe dandruff. In order to treat dandruff brought on by fungal infections, doctors usually prescribe antifungal medications like ciclopirox and ketoconazole. By focusing on the underlying fungal development on the scalp, these drugs successfully lessen flakiness and irritation.

To prevent any possible negative effects, it is imperative to adhere to the recommended dosage and time frame.

Another family of prescription drugs used to treat dandruff include corticosteroids. These anti-inflammatory drugs relieve itching and flaking of the scalp by lowering inflammation and regulating the immune system. Topical corticosteroid creams and solutions are frequently prescribed, however extended use may have negative effects, highlighting the need for medical care.

Light-Based Treatment

An sophisticated dandruff treatment approach called light therapy, sometimes referred to as phototherapy, involves exposing the patient to particular light wavelengths in order to address underlying causes of the condition. UV radiation is commonly used in phototherapy for dandruff and has been shown to be good to the scalp.

Phototherapy for Eczema:

Phototherapy is the administration of UV radiation under regulated conditions, which has the ability to suppress the growth of Malassezia yeast, a common cause of dandruff. A dermatologist oversees the administration of this therapy and decides on the proper length and level of light exposure. It has been demonstrated that UV light lowers inflammation and controls skin cell turnover, all of which improve the environment on the scalp.

Benefits And Drawbacks Of Phototherapy

Although phototherapy is a promising advanced treatment for dandruff, it is important to weigh its benefits and potential downsides. One of the main advantages is that it works well to address the underlying causes of dandruff, giving some people long-lasting relief. Furthermore, light treatment is often well tolerated and non-invasive.

But there are drawbacks to using light therapy to treat dandruff.

Extended or overexposure to ultraviolet radiation can cause sunburn and raise the risk of developing skin cancer, among other negative skin effects. Moreover, phototherapy may not be widely available and may need visits to specialized clinics; additionally, treatment costs may be a major consideration.

In summary, sophisticated dandruff therapies, like prescription drugs and laser therapy, provide focused relief for people with severe symptoms of this scalp ailment. Even if these methods can be relieving, it's important to assess the benefits and drawbacks, taking into account any potential negative effects as well as the practical aspects of each treatment choice. Those looking for cutting-edge dandruff treatments should speak with a medical expert to figure out the best course of action given their unique situation and medical background.

CHAPTER EIGHT
AVOIDING RECURRENCE
OF DANDRUFF

Long-Term tactics: Adopting thorough long-term tactics is necessary for dandruff prevention.

The implementation of efficient maintenance procedures is essential. This entails incorporating the proper methods of cleaning and moisturizing into one's hair care routine. Malassezia yeast, a frequent cause of dandruff, cannot grow out of control on the scalp when it is regularly and gently cleansed using anti-dandruff shampoos. Furthermore, a key factor in the long-term prevention of dandruff is the selection of hair care products. Choosing fragrance-free and hypoallergenic products reduces the possibility of irritating substances that worsen dandruff.

Tracking Triggers: In order to stop dandruff from recurring, it is critical to recognize and keep an eye on triggers.

People need to recognize the things that make their dandruff worse and take proactive steps to deal with them. Hormonal abnormalities, nutritional variables, and stress are common triggers.

To successfully reduce these triggers, dietary changes, stress management practices, and hormone regulation procedures might be used. Environmental aspects should also be taken into account, such as vulnerability to severe weather. People can drastically lower the chance of dandruff recurrence by being watchful and eliminating triggers.

How To Get A Healthy Scalp

Balancing the Scalp Microbiome: Keeping the scalp microbiome in check is essential to having a healthy scalp and avoiding dandruff. A variety of bacteria can be found living on the scalp, and an imbalance in this microbiome may lead to the development of dandruff. Hair care products that contain probiotics and prebiotics can help to maintain a balanced microbial environment on the scalp.

By promoting the development of advantageous microorganisms, these products aid in controlling the population of Malassezia yeast. By supporting the health of the scalp, incorporating these microbiome-friendly products into regular hair care routines will help prevent dandruff.

Frequent Check-Ups: For individuals hoping to stop dandruff from recurring, routine check-ups with dermatologists or other medical specialists with expertise in scalp health are crucial.

These experts are able to evaluate the patient's scalp condition, spot possible problems, and suggest preventative measures that are specific to the patient. Frequent exams also make it easier to identify any developing scalp issues early on and take immediate action. Dermatological assistance makes sure that each person receives information that is specific to their own scalp characteristics and causes of dandruff.

Routine check-ups and other proactive healthcare practices are essential to establishing and preserving a healthy scalp.

CONCLUSION

The prevention of dandruff is a complex process that includes identifying causes, prioritizing scalp health, and implementing long-term methods. Effective dandruff prevention starts with maintenance practices, such using hypoallergenic hair care products and routinely washing with the right anti-dandruff solutions.

Long-term effectiveness in preventing dandruff recurrence also depends on keeping an eye on and managing triggers, which include stress, food, hormone imbalances, and environmental variables.

The utilization of probiotic and prebiotic-containing products is essential for maintaining the delicate balance of the scalp microbiome, which is necessary for achieving a healthy scalp. Scheduling routine examinations with medical specialists who focus on scalp health guarantees individualized treatment and early identification of possible problems. By integrating these components into a thorough strategy, people can experience a healthier scalp and greatly lower the chance of dandruff recurrence. Maintaining good scalp health requires adopting these preventive strategies into everyday routines, as current research continues to reveal insights into the complex dynamics of dandruff.